Turning Stress and Anxiety Around

A Comprehensive and Practical Approach to Discovering and Harnessing the Positives of Stressful Situations

Oswald Albert Harrison

Foreword

In a world that constantly demands more from us—whether through professional pressures, personal challenges, or the myriad expectations that define our modern lives—it's easy to feel overwhelmed. Anxiety and stress have become near-constant companions, often perceived as formidable barriers to our happiness and success. Yet, what if we could change that narrative? What if these very forces, which seem to weigh us down, could be transformed into powerful allies in our quest for growth and fulfillment?

This is not just a book—it's a revelation. It invites you to embark on a transformative journey where stress and anxiety are no longer adversaries but partners in your personal evolution. This book is a beacon of hope, offering a fresh perspective on how to harness the energy of stress and anxiety for your advantage.

Within these pages, you will discover the alchemy of turning life's most daunting challenges into opportunities for profound growth. From understanding the intricate dance between mind and body to applying groundbreaking psychological principles, this book equips you with the tools to not only manage stress but to embrace it as a catalyst for change. The integration of real-life stories and case studies provides a vivid roadmap, demonstrating how individuals from all walks of life have turned their struggles into stepping stones toward success.

Each chapter is a carefully crafted guide, leading you through the process of reframing adversity and building resilience. You will learn practical strategies and insights that are both accessible and transformative. The journey ahead will challenge your perceptions and inspire you to see stress not as an obstacle but as a powerful tool for achieving your goals.

As you delve into this book, you will find that the path to mastering stress and anxiety is not a solitary one. The wisdom shared here is drawn from a tapestry of expert insights, personal triumphs, and innovative approaches. This foreword is a call to action: to embrace the principles and practices outlined within, to commit to your personal growth, and to recognize that stress, when approached with the right mindset, can be a profound force for positive change.

Welcome to a new way of understanding and harnessing the power of stress. Prepare to be inspired, challenged, and empowered. The journey of turning stress and anxiety around begins now, and the potential it unlocks is boundless.

Table of contents

Introduction.

In our fast-paced world, stress and anxiety often feel like inevitable companions. Yet, they hold the potential to be transformed into powerful catalysts for personal growth and success. "Turning Stress and Anxiety Around: A Comprehensive and Practical Approach to Discovering and Harnessing the Positives of Stressful Situations" is crafted to guide you through this transformative journey. This book offers not just relief but a new perspective on stress, showing how it can be harnessed for positive change.

This book is meticulously crafted and thoughtfully curated into five distinct parts, each designed to provide a comprehensive and insightful exploration of turning stress and anxiety into opportunities for growth.

The first part delves into the fundamental nature of stress and anxiety. We begin by defining these concepts and exploring the intricate mind-body connection that amplifies their impact. The scientific insights provided lay the groundwork for understanding how stress functions in our lives. This section also introduces the reframing process, where adversity is viewed as an opportunity for growth. By examining mindset shifts, emotional intelligence, and practical techniques through compelling case studies, you will learn to view stress as a springboard for positive change.

The second part presents a deep dive into the psychological frameworks that underpin stress management. Here, you will explore key theories of stress and performance and see how these theories can be practically applied to enhance well-being. The principles of positive psychology are discussed in depth, revealing how they can transform stress into a tool for personal development. This section emphasizes integrating psychological insights into daily life, enabling you to develop effective personal strategies and adapt them for long-term success.

The third part equips you with actionable techniques to manage stress and boost productivity. From cognitive restructuring and journaling to relaxation exercises, this part provides a toolkit for daily stress relief. You'll discover productivity hacks like the Pomodoro Technique and the Eisenhower Matrix, designed to help you manage your time and tasks more efficiently. The focus on goal setting and achievement guides you through creating clear action plans, overcoming obstacles, and reflecting on progress, ensuring you make the most of your newfound strategies.

The fourth part brings theory into reality with inspiring profiles of individuals who have turned stress into success. Through engaging interviews with experts and achievers from various fields, you will gain diverse perspectives on stress management. This section highlights how these individuals have applied the principles discussed earlier and offers actionable takeaways that you can adapt to your own life. The real-world applications provide both inspiration and practical advice, demonstrating the transformative power of stress when approached with the right mindset.

The concluding part of this book entails integrating stress management techniques with broader wellness practices. Here, the focus is on creating a balanced routine that includes exercise, nutrition, and sleep. Achieving work-life balance is discussed in detail, offering strategies to avoid burnout and maintain harmony between personal and professional life. This section also emphasizes the importance of long-term lifestyle changes, helping you build resilience and develop sustainable health habits that will support ongoing stress management.

Through this book, you will embark on a journey of turning stress and anxiety into opportunities for growth and success. Each part is meticulously designed to build on the previous one, offering a comprehensive guide to transforming challenges into triumphs. Discover how to harness the positives of stress and unlock your potential for a more balanced and fulfilling life.

PART 1: UNDER-STANDING AND TRANSFORMING STRESS AND ANXIETY

Chapter 1

Understanding Stress and Its Impact

Stress is a fundamental aspect of human experience, influencing various facets of our lives. Understanding its nature and effects is crucial for harnessing its potential for growth.

What is Stress and Anxiety?

Stress and anxiety, though often used interchangeably, refer to distinct concepts. Stress is a response to external pressures, often triggered by specific events or situations. It can be acute or chronic and varies in intensity and duration. Anxiety, on the other hand, is a more persistent state characterized by excessive worry or apprehension, often without a specific trigger.

Stress involves physiological and psychological responses to perceived threats or challenges. It includes a range of reactions from mild discomfort to severe distress. Stressors, or the sources of stress, can be internal (e.g., self-imposed expectations) or external (e.g., work deadlines, personal conflicts). Understanding the distinction between acute stress, which is short-term and typically linked to immediate challenges, and chronic stress, which persists over a long period and can lead to significant health issues, is crucial for managing stress effectively.

Anxiety is often characterized by feelings of unease, dread, or apprehension. It can manifest as generalized anxiety disorder (GAD), panic attacks, or social anxiety, among other forms. Unlike stress, which may have an identifiable cause, anxiety can occur without a specific trigger and is often associated with a heightened state of alertness and concern about potential future threats.

Although stress and anxiety often overlap, stress is usually a reaction to a specific event or situation, while anxiety can be a more enduring and generalized state. Understanding this distinction is essential for addressing each effectively.

The Mind-Body Connection

The interplay between the mind and body plays a crucial role in stress response. When faced with a stressor, the body undergoes a series of physiological changes designed to prepare for a "fight or flight" response. This includes the release of stress hormones such as cortisol and adrenaline, which can impact various bodily systems.

Physiological Impact

Stress affects numerous physiological systems. The cardiovascular system may experience increased heart rate and blood pressure. The immune system can be suppressed, leading to a greater susceptibility to illness. Muscles may tense up, contributing to physical discomfort or pain. Chronic stress can exacerbate these effects, leading to long-term health issues such as cardiovascular disease, gastrointestinal problems, and chronic pain conditions.

Mental and Emotional Impacts

Psychologically, stress can affect cognitive functions, such as memory and concentration. It can lead to emotional responses such as irritability, depression, or anxiety. The ongoing stress response can create a cycle where the mental burden exacerbates physical symptoms, and vice versa.

Long-Term Impact on Well-being

Chronic stress can contribute to the development of mental health disorders such as depression and anxiety disorders. Understanding the connection between stress and mental well-being is crucial for developing effective coping strategies.

The Role of Stress in Daily Life

Stress is an inevitable part of daily life, influencing various domains, including work, relationships, and personal wellbeing. Understanding how stress operates within these contexts can provide insights into managing it effectively.

Stress can both positively and negatively affect productivity. Short-term stress may enhance focus and performance, while chronic stress can lead to burnout and decreased efficiency. Identifying the optimal level of stress for productivity is crucial for achieving balance.

1. In the Workplace

Stress in the workplace can stem from factors such as high demands, tight deadlines, and interpersonal conflicts. It can affect job performance, satisfaction, and overall well-being. Effective stress management strategies, such as time management, relaxation techniques, and seeking support, are essential for maintaining workplace health.

2. In Personal Relationships

Stress can impact relationships by increasing irritability, reducing communication, and causing conflicts. Building strong, supportive relationships and employing communication strategies can help manage stress and strengthen personal connections. Understanding how stress affects interpersonal dynamics can help individuals develop strategies to maintain healthy relationships.

3. Personal Well-being

Stress can influence overall well-being by affecting physical health, emotional stability, and life satisfaction but when managed effectively, it can be a catalyst for personal growth. It can drive individuals to develop new skills, overcome challenges, and achieve goals. Embracing stress as a motivator and learning to adapt to stressors can contribute to long-term personal development. By recognizing the multifaceted impact of stress, individuals can better address its effects and seek appropriate support.

Understanding stress and its impact is the first step toward transforming it into a productive force. This foundational knowledge sets the stage for applying psychological theories and practical strategies in subsequent chapters.

Chapter 2

Scientific Insights into Stress

Understanding the scientific basis of stress is essential for developing effective strategies to manage it. There are key scientific researches on stress, examining its physiological, cognitive, and emotional impacts and we explore them in this chapter. By grounding stress management techniques in scientific research, we can better appreciate how to harness stress for personal and professional growth.

The Biopsychosocial Model of Stress

The biopsychosocial model provides a comprehensive framework for understanding stress. It integrates biological, psychological, and social factors to explain how stress affects individuals and their health.

Biological Factors

Stress triggers physiological responses that prepare the body to deal with perceived threats. The autonomic nervous system (ANS) activates the fight-or-flight response, leading to the release of stress hormones such as cortisol and adrenaline. Prolonged activation of this response can contribute to health issues like hypertension, diabetes, and weakened immune function.

Psychological Factors

Psychological factors, including perception and cognition, play a critical role in stress. How individuals perceive and interpret stressors affects their emotional and physiological responses. Cognitive appraisals—evaluations of the threat or challenge posed by stressors—determine the intensity and impact of stress.

Social Factors

Social support and environmental factors influence how stress is experienced and managed. Supportive relationships, social networks, and community resources can mitigate the negative effects of stress. Conversely, social isolation and adverse life events can exacerbate stress.

Studies have demonstrated that individuals with strong social support networks experience less physiological reactivity to stress and report better mental health outcomes. Conversely, those with high levels of perceived stress and low social support are at greater risk for adverse health outcomes.

Stress and the Nervous System

Stress impacts the nervous system, with significant implications for overall health and well-being. Understanding these effects can aid in developing effective stress management strategies.

The Autonomic Nervous System (ANS)

The ANS regulates involuntary physiological functions such as heart rate, respiration, and digestion. During stress, the sympathetic branch of the ANS is activated, leading to increased heart rate, blood pressure, and energy mobilization. Chronic stress can lead to sustained activation of the sympathetic nervous system, contributing to cardiovascular problems and other health issues.

The Hypothalamic-Pituitary-Adrenal (HPA) Axis

The HPA axis plays a key role in the stress response by regulating the release of cortisol. Cortisol helps manage energy levels and modulates immune responses. Chronic stress can lead to dysregulation of the HPA axis, resulting in elevated cortisol levels, which can contribute to metabolic disorders, immune suppression, and mood disturbances.

Neuroplasticity and Stress

Neuroplasticity refers to the brain's ability to reorganize and adapt in response to experiences. Chronic stress can affect neuroplasticity, leading to changes in brain structure and function. Stress-related changes in brain regions such as the amygdala and prefrontal cortex can impact emotional regulation, memory, and cognitive function.

Research shows that chronic stress is associated with structural changes in the brain, including reduced hippocampal volume and increased amygdala activation. These changes can affect memory, emotional regulation, and cognitive performance.

Stress and Cognitive Function

Stress influences cognitive processes, including attention, memory, and decision-making amongst others. Understanding these effects is crucial for developing strategies to manage stress and enhance cognitive function.

Attention and Focus

Acute stress can improve attention and focus by increasing arousal and alertness. However, chronic stress can impair attention by leading to distractibility and difficulty concentrating. Research indicates that high levels of stress are associated with reduced cognitive flexibility and attention deficits.

Memory

Stress affects memory consolidation and retrieval. Acute stress can enhance memory formation for emotionally salient events, but chronic stress can impair both short-term and long-term memory. Stress-related changes in brain regions such as the hippocampus can contribute to memory problems.

Decision-Making

Stress influences decision-making processes, often leading to riskier or more impulsive choices. High levels of stress can impair judgment and problem-solving abilities, affecting decision-making in both personal and professional contexts.

Apart from these, stress also affects emotional regulation, leading to increased emotional reactivity, mood swings, and difficulties in managing emotions. Studies have shown that chronic stress can exacerbate symptoms of anxiety and depression, impacting overall mental health.

While chronic stress can hinder creativity, moderate levels of stress can stimulate creative thinking by fostering problem-solving and innovation. Research suggests that stress can lead to increased cognitive flexibility and idea generation when managed effectively.

Stress and Emotional Well-Being

The relationship between stress and emotional well-being is complex and multifaceted. Stress can have both positive and negative effects on emotions, depending on its intensity and duration.

Emotional Responses to Stress

Stress can trigger a range of emotional responses, including anxiety, irritability, and depression. Acute stress may lead to heightened emotional arousal, while chronic stress can contribute to persistent negative emotions and mood disorders.

Stress and Coping Strategies

Effective coping strategies can mitigate the negative emotional impact of stress. Techniques such as mindfulness, cognitive-behavioral therapy (CBT), and relaxation exercises can help individuals manage their emotional responses to stress.

Research indicates that mindfulness and CBT are effective in reducing stress and improving emotional well-being. Studies have shown that mindfulness-based interventions can reduce symptoms of anxiety and depression, while CBT can help individuals develop adaptive coping skills.

Implications for Stress Management

Understanding the scientific basis of stress provides valuable insights for developing effective stress management strategies. By addressing the biological, psychological, and social factors that contribute to stress, individuals can implement targeted interventions to improve their overall well-being.

Effective stress management strategies should consider the physiological, cognitive, and emotional impacts of stress. Techniques such as mindfulness, cognitive restructuring, and social support can be integrated into daily life to enhance stress resilience and overall health.

Recognizing individual differences in stress responses and coping mechanisms is essential for personalized stress management. Tailoring strategies to personal needs and preferences can improve one's effectiveness and support long-term well-being.

By exploring the scientific underpinnings of stress, this chapter provides a comprehensive understanding of how stress affects the body and mind. The insights gained from scientific research offer a foundation for developing practical strategies to manage stress effectively, setting the stage for more detailed exploration in subsequent chapters.

Chapter 3

The Reframing Process

Transforming stress from a detrimental force into a positive driver for growth involves reframing how we perceive and manage stress and reframing stress often involves a change in our perception of it from a source of threat to an opportunity for growth. By mastering these reframing strategies, individuals can harness stress effectively and enhance their overall well-being.

Mindset Shifts

The way we perceive stress significantly influences how it affects us. Transforming stress from a perceived threat to a challenge requires a fundamental shift in mindset.

Viewing stress as a threat often leads to a stress response characterized by anxiety, avoidance, and impaired performance. Conversely, seeing stress as a challenge can enhance motivation, focus, and resilience. This shift involves recognizing stress as an opportunity to grow and achieve, rather than as an insurmountable obstacle.

Adopting a growth mindset, as proposed by psychologist Carol Dweck, involves believing that abilities and intelligence can be developed through effort and learning. This mindset encourages individuals to embrace challenges, learn from failures, and persist in the face of adversity, ultimately transforming stress into a tool for personal growth.

Techniques for fostering a growth mindset include setting challenging yet achievable goals, seeking feedback, and reflecting on past experiences. By framing stress as a pathway to growth, individuals can enhance their capacity to manage stress effectively and achieve their objectives.

Emotional Intelligence

Emotional intelligence (EI) involves understanding and managing one's own emotions, as well as recognizing and influencing the emotions of others. Developing EI can turn stress and anxiety into drivers for personal development.

Being aware of one's emotional responses to stress is the first step in managing it effectively. Self-awareness allows individuals to recognize stress triggers, understand their emotional reactions, and make informed decisions about how to address them.

Self-regulation involves managing emotions in a healthy and constructive manner. Techniques such as mindfulness, deep breathing, and cognitive restructuring can help individuals control their emotional responses and prevent stress from becoming overwhelming.

Emotional intelligence also includes the ability to empathize with others and navigate social interactions effectively. Building strong relationships and effective communication skills can help individuals manage stress in interpersonal contexts and create supportive environments.

To enhance EI, individuals can practice mindfulness, engage in reflective journaling, and seek feedback from others. Developing EI not only helps in managing personal stress but also improves interactions and relationships with others.

PART 2: PSYCHOLOGICA L THEORIES AND STRESS MANAGEMENT

Chapter 4

Theoretical Foundations of Stress

Psychological theories offer valuable insights into how stress affects performance and well-being. Now we explore some foundational theories related to stress, providing a framework for understanding how these theories can be applied to manage stress effectively and enhance productivity.

Key Psychological Theories on Stress

Several psychological theories provide a framework for understanding stress and its effects on behavior and performance. Some of the most influential theories include:

The Yerkes-Dodson Law

The Yerkes-Dodson Law provides a foundational understanding of the relationship between stress and performance. This theory posits an inverted U-shaped relationship between stress and performance and suggests that performance increases with physiological or mental arousal (stress) up to an optimal point. Beyond this point, additional stress can lead to decreased performance.

Research indicates that each individual has an optimal stress level that maximizes their performance. This level varies depending on the nature of the task and the individual's baseline stress tolerance. Tasks that are complex or require higher cognitive function benefit from lower to moderate stress levels, while tasks requiring physical exertion may benefit from higher stress levels.

To apply this theory, one must first identify their personal optimal stress levels through experimentation and self-assessment. Techniques to manage stress level include setting realistic goals, prioritizing tasks, and using stress reduction techniques to maintain performance within the optimal range.

Stress Inoculation Theory

Stress Inoculation Theory (SIT) developed by Donald Meichenbaum, proposes that individuals can be trained to manage stress through gradual exposure and coping strategies. This theory emphasizes that exposure to manageable stressors can build resilience and improve stress management capabilities.

SIT involves exposing individuals to controlled and manageable levels of stress to build tolerance and coping skills. This process helps individuals become better equipped to handle higher levels of stress when they arise. Gradual exposure can include simulations, role-playing, and controlled challenges.

As individuals are exposed to stress, they learn and practice coping strategies to manage their responses. These strategies may include problem-solving techniques, relaxation exercises, and cognitive reframing. The goal is to build a repertoire of effective coping mechanisms that can be employed in real-world stress situations.

One can implement SIT by gradually increasing exposure to stressors and practicing coping techniques in a controlled environment. This approach can enhance resilience and improve the ability to handle higher levels of stress in various life domains.

Cognitive Appraisal Theory

Cognitive appraisal theory, developed by Richard Lazarus, focuses on how individuals evaluate and interpret stressors. This evaluation determines the emotional and physiological responses to stress.

The initial assessment of whether a stressor is relevant to one's well-being is called the primary appraisal. In this stage, individuals determine if the stressor is a threat, challenge, or benign. For example, receiving a work deadline might be appraised as a threat if it feels overwhelming or as a challenge if it is seen as an opportunity for growth.

The subsequent evaluation of available resources and coping mechanisms to deal with the stressor is called the secondary appraisal. This stage involves assessing whether one has the necessary resources and skills to handle the stressor effectively. For instance, evaluating whether one can manage the workload through time management skills or seeking support from colleagues.

The process of reassessing the situation after the initial response is known as the reappraisal. Reappraisal allows for adjustment of strategies and coping mechanisms based on new information or changes in the situation. It involves re-evaluating the stressor and one's response to it, which can lead to a shift in perspective and reduced stress.

The Stress-Diathesis Model

This model suggests that stress interacts with individual vulnerabilities to influence mental health outcomes. It posits that stress alone may not lead to psychological disorders, but when combined with pre-existing vulnerabilities (such as genetic predispositions or early life experiences), it can contribute to the development of mental health conditions.

Understanding this interaction can help in developing targeted stress management strategies for individuals at risk. This model emphasizes the need for personalized approaches to stress management, considering both stress exposure and individual susceptibilities.

To apply the Stress-Diathesis Model, one must develop strategies to address personal vulnerabilities by incorporating preventative measures and tailored interventions. This might include targeted therapy, stress management training, and lifestyle adjustments to mitigate the impact of stress on mental health.

The Fight-or-Flight Response

Proposed by Walter Cannon, the fight-or-flight response describes the physiological changes that occur when an individual perceives a threat. This includes the activation of the autonomic nervous system, leading to increased heart rate, elevated adrenaline levels, and heightened alertness.

Understanding this response helps in recognizing how acute stress can temporarily enhance performance and focus, but can also lead to detrimental effects if prolonged.

Techniques to manage the physiological impacts of stress include deep breathing exercises, progressive muscle relaxation, and mindfulness practices. These methods help counteract the physiological arousal associated with the fight-or-flight response and promote a state of calm.

Chapter 5

Positive Psychology and Stress Management

Positive psychology focuses on enhancing well-being and personal growth by leveraging positive emotions, strengths, and experiences. This chapter explores how principles of positive psychology can be applied to manage stress effectively, transforming stress from a challenge into an opportunity for growth.

Principles of Positive Psychology

Positive psychology emphasizes the study and promotion of positive aspects of human experience. Key principles include:

1. **Finding Meaning in Adversity**

One of the central tenets of positive psychology is finding meaning in challenging experiences. Research shows that individuals who perceive stress as an opportunity for growth or a meaningful challenge are more likely to experience positive outcomes. This perspective shift can turn stressful situations into opportunities for learning and development. Identify the potential benefits and learning opportunities within stressful experiences. This involves reflecting on how challenges can lead to personal growth and improved skills. Techniques such as journaling and cognitive reframing can aid in this process.

2. Developing a Growth Mindset

A growth mindset, as proposed by Carol Dweck, involves viewing challenges and failures as opportunities for development rather than as threats. This mindset encourages individuals to embrace stress as a catalyst for personal and professional growth. This can be done by adopting exercises and strategies that embrace challenges, such as setting stretch goals and viewing setbacks as learning opportunities.

3. Leveraging Strengths

Positive psychology also focuses on identifying and using personal strengths. By leveraging these strengths in the face of stress, one can improve their ability to cope with challenges and achieve their goals. One can identify their personal strengths through tools like strengths assessments or self-reflection exercises. These strengths can be used when facing stress, such as applying problem-solving skills, creativity, or perseverance to overcome challenges.

4. Cultivating Positive Emotions

Positive emotions, such as gratitude, joy, and hope, are integral to positive psychology. Cultivating these emotions can counterbalance the effects of stress, enhancing overall well-being and resilience. Practices for cultivating positive emotions, such as gratitude exercises, mindfulness practices, and engaging in activities that bring joy can be implemented. These practices can help offset the negative effects of stress and contribute to a more balanced emotional state.

Practical Techniques and Tools

Integrating positive psychology principles into stress management involves practical techniques and strategies that enhance well-being and performance. Some of those techniques include:

1. Gratitude Practices

Gratitude exercises, such as keeping a gratitude journal or regularly reflecting on things one is thankful for, have been shown to reduce stress and increase overall well-being. These practices help shift focus from stressors to positive aspects of life, fostering a more optimistic outlook.

2. Optimism Training

Training in optimism involves developing a positive outlook and reframing negative thoughts. Techniques such as cognitive restructuring and positive affirmations can help individuals challenge and change negative thought patterns, turning stress into a source of motivation.

3. Mindfulness and Meditation

Mindfulness practices, including meditation and mindful breathing, are central to positive psychology. These techniques help individuals stay present and manage stress more effectively by reducing rumination and enhancing emotional regulation.

4. Strengths-Based Goal Setting

Setting goals based on personal strengths aligns with positive psychology principles. By focusing on areas where they excel, individuals can create achievable and motivating goals that enhance their ability to manage stress and achieve success.

5. Positive Visualization

Practice positive visualization techniques, such as imagining successful outcomes and focusing on desired results. Visualization can boost confidence and reduce anxiety associated with stress.

Integrating Positive Psychology into Stress Management

To effectively integrate positive psychology principles into stress management, consider the following steps:

Create a personal plan that incorporates gratitude practices, optimism training, mindfulness, and strengths-based goal setting. Tailor the plan to your needs and preferences, ensuring it aligns with personal values and goals. Also, regularly practicing these techniques as consistent application will reinforce the benefits and enhance stress management.

Regularly assess the effectiveness of positive psychology techniques in managing stress. Use tools such as self-assessment questionnaires and progress journals to track improvements and adjust strategies as needed.

Engage in communities or support groups that practice positive psychology principles. Sharing experiences and learning from others can enhance the effectiveness of stress management strategies and provide additional motivation.

Stay informed about new developments in positive psychology and stress management. Continuously adapt and refine techniques based on personal experiences and emerging research to maintain and improve stress management practices.

By exploring the principles of positive psychology and their application to stress management, we can obtain a comprehensive understanding of how to leverage positive emotions and strengths to transform stress into a powerful force for personal growth. The insights and techniques offered will help manage stress effectively and enhance overall well-being.

Chapter 6

Integrating Psychological Insights into Daily Life

Incorporating psychological theories and models into everyday routines can enhance stress management and promote personal growth. This chapter focuses on translating theoretical insights into practical strategies that can be seamlessly integrated into daily life. It provides actionable steps for developing personal strategies, ensuring long-term integration, and continuously monitoring and adjusting methods for optimal effectiveness.

Translating Theory into Practice

Applying psychological theories to real-life scenarios requires understanding how to translate theoretical concepts into practical actions.

Begin by summarizing key psychological theories relevant to stress management, such as the Yerkes-Dodson Law, the fight-or-flight response, and positive psychology principles. Ensure a clear understanding of these concepts to effectively apply them in daily life.

Identify specific ways to implement these theories in everyday routines. For instance, use the Yerkes-Dodson Law to set achievable stress levels that enhance productivity, or apply positive psychology principles by integrating gratitude practices and optimism training into daily habits.

Develop a customized plan that incorporates these practical applications. Tailor the strategies to individual preferences and needs, ensuring they align with personal goals and lifestyle. This might involve creating a daily schedule that balances work and relaxation or setting specific goals based on strengths.

Developing Personal Strategies

Personal strategies for managing stress and enhancing productivity should be grounded in psychological insights.

Start by identifying individual stressors and understanding how they affect daily life. This might involve tracking stress levels, noting patterns, and pinpointing specific triggers.

Choose techniques based on psychological theories that address personal stressors. For example, if stress is related to performance, use the Yerkes-Dodson Law to set optimal stress levels and employ time management techniques to maintain balance.

Establish mechanisms for ongoing feedback to evaluate the effectiveness of the strategies. Regular self-assessment, journaling, or feedback from a mentor can help track progress and make necessary adjustments.

Be prepared to modify strategies based on personal experiences and evolving stress levels. Flexibility is key to maintaining effectiveness and adapting to changing circumstances.

Long-Term Integration

Integrating psychological insights into long-term stress management involves embedding strategies into daily routines and ensuring sustainability.

Develop routines that incorporate stress management techniques and psychological principles. This might involve establishing daily practices such as mindfulness meditation, goal setting, and regular exercise.

Focus on building and maintaining habits that support stress management. Techniques such as habit stacking, where new habits are linked to existing ones, can facilitate long-term integration.

Implement systems for tracking progress over time. This could include maintaining a stress management journal, using apps for goal tracking, or setting periodic review dates to assess progress and make adjustments.

Regularly evaluate the effectiveness of integrated strategies. Reflect on what is working well and identify areas for improvement. This ongoing evaluation helps in refining strategies and maintaining effectiveness.

Monitoring and Adjusting

Continuous monitoring and adjustment are crucial for effective stress management. This section outlines how to stay on track and make necessary changes.

Schedule regular check-ins to assess stress levels and the effectiveness of strategies. This might involve weekly reviews or monthly assessments to ensure that strategies remain relevant and effective.

Engage with support networks, such as mentors, coaches, or peer groups, for feedback and guidance. Support systems can provide valuable insights and encouragement for maintaining effective practices.

Be prepared to adapt strategies in response to changes in personal circumstances or stress levels. Flexibility and openness to change are essential for ongoing success.

Stay informed about new research and developments in psychological theories and stress management techniques. Incorporate new insights and practices to continually enhance stress management strategies.

Coping Strategies

Effective coping strategies are essential for managing stress and enhancing resilience. This section explores various coping mechanisms and their impact on stress.

1. Problem-Focused Coping

This approach involves addressing the root cause of stress directly. It includes strategies such as problem-solving, time management, and seeking support. Problem-focused coping aims to alter the stressor or one's response to it to reduce its impact.

2. Emotion-Focused Coping

This approach involves managing the emotional response to stress rather than addressing the stressor itself. Techniques include mindfulness, relaxation exercises, and emotional expression. Emotion-focused coping helps in regulating emotional reactions and reducing the psychological impact of stress.

3. Adaptive vs. Maladaptive Coping

Adaptive coping strategies, such as positive reframing and seeking social support, contribute to long-term well-being and effective stress management. In contrast, maladaptive strategies, such as avoidance or substance abuse, can exacerbate stress and lead to negative outcomes. Understanding the difference between adaptive and maladaptive coping is crucial for developing effective stress management techniques.

Practical exercises and activities can help in developing effective coping skills. Techniques such as stress journaling, role-playing scenarios, and mindfulness practices can enhance coping abilities and build resilience.

Integrating psychological insights into daily life involves a continuous process of applying theories, developing personal strategies, and making adjustments as needed. The principles and techniques outlined in this chapter provide a foundation for transforming theoretical insights into practical, actionable strategies that promote long-term success.

PART 3:

PRACTICAL

STRATEGIES

AND

EFFECTIVE

TECHNIQUES

Chapter 7

Essential Stress Management Techniques

Effective stress management requires practical tools and techniques that individuals can incorporate into their daily routines. Each technique is explained in detail, with practical guidance on how to apply them to achieve optimal stress reduction and enhance overall well-being.

Cognitive Restructuring

Cognitive restructuring involves identifying and challenging negative thought patterns that contribute to stress. By altering these thought patterns, individuals can reduce their stress responses and improve their emotional resilience.

Begin by recognizing common negative thoughts and cognitive distortions. Cognitive distortions are inaccurate or exaggerated thought patterns that can heighten stress. Common distortions include all-or-nothing thinking, catastrophizing, and overgeneralization. Recognizing these distortions is the first step in cognitive restructuring. Use self-monitoring tools, such as thought records or journaling, to identify these patterns.

Employ techniques such as thought recording, where individuals write down their negative thoughts and examine evidence for and against them. Learn to challenge these negative thoughts. Use techniques such as Socratic questioning to explore alternative, more balanced perspectives. For instance, if you think, "I always mess up," challenge this by listing instances where you succeeded.

Replace negative thoughts with more balanced and realistic ones. Cognitive-behavioral therapy (CBT) techniques, such as cognitive challenging and reappraisal, can help reframe these thoughts in a more balanced and realistic manner. Practice affirmations and positive self-talk to reinforce these new perspectives. For example, instead of "I can't handle this," try, "I've managed similar challenges before, and I can handle this one too."

Integrate cognitive restructuring into daily routines by setting aside time for reflective practices, such as journaling or thought records. Use cognitive restructuring techniques during stressful situations to challenge and reframe negative thoughts, reducing their impact on stress levels.

Journaling for Stress Relief

Journaling provides a structured way to process and manage stress by allowing individuals to express their thoughts and feelings. This technique can help identify stressors, track progress, and gain insights into personal stress patterns.

Explore different types of journaling, including expressive writing, where individuals freely write about their emotions and experiences, and structured journaling, which involves prompts or specific questions to guide reflection. Both types can be effective for stress relief.

Keep a gratitude journal to regularly record things you are thankful for. Reflecting on positive aspects of life can shift focus away from stressors and foster a more optimistic outlook. Use reflective journaling to explore daily experiences and emotions. Write about stressors, how you managed them, and what you learned. This practice helps identify patterns and triggers, enabling more effective stress management.

Maintain an emotion log to track your emotional responses to various situations. Note the intensity and duration of your emotions and any associated thoughts. Analyzing these logs can help in understanding and addressing emotional reactions.

Journaling can reduce stress by providing a safe outlet for emotional expression, helping individuals gain perspective, and identifying patterns in their stress responses. It also fosters mindfulness and self-awareness.

Establish a regular journaling routine, such as daily or weekly sessions. Choose a format that resonates with personal preferences and needs. Incorporate prompts or topics related to current stressors or achievements to guide entries and enhance their effectiveness.

Relaxation Exercises

Relaxation exercises help manage stress by inducing a state of calm and reducing physiological stress responses. Techniques such as deep breathing, progressive muscle relaxation, and guided imagery can be integrated into daily routines for effective stress management.

Deep breathing exercises involve focusing on slow, deep breaths to activate the body's relaxation response. Techniques such as diaphragmatic breathing and 4-7-8 breathing can reduce stress and promote relaxation.

Progressive muscle relaxation (PMR) involves tensing and then relaxing different muscle groups to release physical tension associated with stress. This technique helps individuals become more aware of their bodily stress responses and promotes relaxation.

Guided imagery involves using mental visualization to create a calming and peaceful environment. By focusing on positive or relaxing imagery, individuals can reduce stress and enhance emotional well-being.

Incorporate mindfulness meditation into your routine to cultivate awareness and presence. Practice mindfulness by focusing on your breath, bodily sensations, or a particular object. Regular mindfulness practice can reduce stress and enhance emotional regulation.

Integrate relaxation exercises into daily routines, such as practicing deep breathing before bed or during stressful moments. Set aside specific times for PMR or guided imagery sessions to maintain consistent practice and optimize stress management benefits.

Daily Implementation

Effective stress management techniques require consistent application to be truly beneficial.

Develop a daily or weekly routine that includes stress management practices. Designate specific times for cognitive restructuring, journaling, and relaxation exercises to ensure these techniques become integral parts of daily life. Use reminders or prompts to reinforce the use of stress management techniques. Digital tools, such as calendar alerts or smartphone apps, can help remind individuals to practice these techniques regularly.

Establish realistic and achievable goals for implementing stress management techniques. Start with small, manageable changes and gradually increase your commitment as you become more comfortable with the practices.

Regularly assess the effectiveness of stress management techniques by tracking stress levels and personal experiences. Use journals or self-assessment tools to evaluate progress and make adjustments to techniques as needed. Be flexible and open to modifying techniques based on your evolving needs and circumstances. Experiment with different approaches and adapt them to fit your lifestyle and stress levels.

Focus on building habits around stress management techniques by incorporating them into daily routines and reinforcing their use over time. Celebrate successes and milestones to maintain motivation and commitment to the practices.

Implementing these essential stress management techniques can effectively reduce stress levels and enhance overall well-being. Cognitive restructuring, journaling, and relaxation exercises provide practical tools for managing stress and improving emotional resilience, ensuring a comprehensive approach to stress management.

Chapter 8

Productivity Hacks and Time Management

The focus of this chapter is on enhancing productivity through effective time management and productivity hacks. It provides actionable techniques and strategies that can be implemented to manage time more efficiently and improve overall productivity, especially under stress.

Pomodoro Technique

The Pomodoro Technique is a time management method that promotes sustained focus and productivity by breaking work into intervals traditionally 25 minutes in length, separated by short breaks.. This section explores its principles and applications

The Pomodoro Technique was developed by Francesco Cirillo in the late 1980s. It uses a timer, traditionally set for 25 minutes, called a "Pomodoro," followed by a 5-minute break. After four intervals or Pomodoros, a longer break of 15-30 minutes is taken.

Start by selecting a task you need to complete. Set a timer for 25 minutes and work on the task until the timer rings. Take a 5-minute break to rest and recharge. Repeat this cycle, and after four intervals, take a longer break to refresh.

This method helps manage distractions and maintain focus by creating a sense of urgency. It also prevents burnout by ensuring regular breaks, which can enhance overall productivity and work quality. It helps in managing tasks more effectively and reduces procrastination. Users often find that breaking work into smaller intervals makes it more manageable.

Customize the intervals based on your preferences and the complexity of the tasks. For example, you might choose longer work sessions for more complex tasks or shorter intervals for less demanding ones.

Eisenhower Matrix

The Eisenhower Matrix also known as the Urgent-Important Matrix is a decision-making tool that helps prioritize tasks based on their urgency and importance.

The matrix divides tasks into four quadrants:

1. **Urgent and Important**

Tasks that need immediate attention and are crucial for achieving goals. Handle these tasks first.

2. **Important but Not Urgent**

Tasks that are significant but do not require immediate action. Schedule time for these tasks to prevent them from becoming urgent.

3. Urgent but Not Important

Tasks that demand immediate attention but are not crucial. Delegate these tasks if possible or handle them quickly.

4. Not Urgent and Not Important

Tasks that have little value and do not require immediate attention. Consider eliminating or minimizing these tasks.

List all tasks and categorize them into the four quadrants. Focus on completing tasks in the "Urgent and Important" quadrant first. Schedule time for "Important but Not Urgent" tasks and delegate or minimize "Urgent but Not Important" and "Not Urgent and Not Important" tasks.

The Eisenhower Matrix helps in prioritizing tasks effectively, reducing procrastination, and ensuring that time is spent on high-impact activities. It enhances productivity by focusing on what truly matters and avoiding distractions.

Adjust the categories and prioritization criteria based on your specific goals and responsibilities. Use digital tools or physical planners to track and manage tasks effectively.

Task Batching and Time Blocking

Task batching and time blocking are techniques used to organize and allocate time efficiently for different types of tasks. This section explores these methods and their benefits.

Group similar tasks together and perform them consecutively. For example, batch all email responses or administrative tasks into a specific time block. This reduces the cognitive load of switching between different types of tasks and improves efficiency.

Allocate specific blocks of time in your schedule for focused work on particular tasks or projects. Each block should be dedicated to a single task or activity, with scheduled breaks in between. Use a calendar or planner to set these blocks and stick to the schedule.

Task batching reduces the cognitive load associated with multitasking and helps maintain focus. Time blocking provides structure to the day, making it easier to manage time and avoid procrastination. Both techniques improve productivity and stress management. They also help in setting boundaries and maintaining work-life balance.

Develop a daily or weekly schedule that incorporates task batching and time blocking. Use digital tools or planners to set up your schedule and track your adherence. Regularly review and adjust your approach based on productivity levels and changing priorities.

Creating a Productive Environment

A conducive work environment can significantly impact productivity and a productive environment is crucial for effective time management and stress reduction.

Identify common distractions in your work environment, such as noise, mobile notifications, or clutter by keeping your workplace tidy. Implement strategies to minimize these distractions, such as using noise-canceling headphones, turning off non-essential notifications, or setting clear boundaries with others.

Cultivate a positive mental environment by setting clear goals, maintaining motivation, and practicing mindfulness. Create routines that foster focus and reduce stress, such as starting the day with a planning session or incorporating short mindfulness breaks.

Create a workspace that is inspiring and comfortable. Use elements such as lighting, plants, and motivational items to enhance your work environment. Ensure that your workspace is equipped with the necessary tools and resources for optimal productivity. Optimize your digital workspace by managing notifications, using productivity tools, and organizing files. Implement strategies to reduce digital clutter and avoid interruptions from social media or unrelated online activities.

A well-organized and supportive environment enhances focus, reduces stress, and boosts productivity. It helps in managing time effectively and creates a space where work can be completed efficiently. Regularly assess and update your workspace to ensure it remains conducive to productivity. Make adjustments based on changes in your work style or needs. Experiment with different setups and tools to find what works best for you.

By incorporating these productivity hacks and time management techniques, individuals can enhance their ability to manage tasks, reduce stress, and achieve their goals more effectively. The practical strategies examined can be integrated into daily routines to improve productivity and overall work efficiency.

Chapter 9

Goal Setting and Achievement

This chapter focuses on practical strategies for setting and achieving goals, with an emphasis on overcoming obstacles and maintaining progress. It provides individuals with the tools and techniques needed to transform their aspirations into actionable plans and ensures they stay motivated and focused on their objectives.

SMART Goals

The SMART framework is a widely used method for setting clear and achievable goals. The components of the SMART criteria and guidance on how to apply them effectively are outlined below

1. Specific

Goals should be clear and specific. Define what you want to achieve, why it is important, and who is involved. Avoid vague statements; be as precise as possible. For instance, instead of setting a goal like "get fit," specify "run a 5K in under 30 minutes."

2. Measurable

Establish criteria to measure progress and determine when the goal has been achieved. Include quantifiable elements such as numbers, dates, or milestones. For example, "increase sales by 15% within six months" provides a clear measure of success.

3. Achievable

Goals should be realistic and attainable. Consider the resources and constraints you have, and set goals that are challenging yet achievable. Assess whether you have the necessary skills, time, and resources to accomplish the goal.

4. Relevant

Ensure the goal aligns with broader objectives and values. It should be meaningful and relevant to your long-term plans or career aspirations. For example, a goal to "complete a certification course relevant to your field" should align with your career advancement plans.

5. Time-bound

Set a deadline for achieving the goal. A specific time frame creates a sense of urgency and helps maintain focus. For instance, "finish the project by the end of the quarter" provides a clear deadline for completion.

The SMART framework helps in creating well-defined goals, ensuring that they are actionable and measurable. It enhances motivation by setting clear expectations and deadlines, and provides a structured approach to achieving objectives.

Adjust the SMART criteria based on your personal needs and circumstances. Regularly review and revise goals as needed to stay aligned with changing priorities and situations.

Action Plans and Milestones

Action plans and milestones are essential for breaking down goals into manageable steps and tracking progress. Outlined below is the guidance to creating effective action plans and setting milestones to ensure steady progress towards goal achievement

Action Plan

Develop a detailed action plan outlining the specific steps needed to achieve each goal. Break down the goal into smaller, actionable tasks and assign deadlines for each task. An action plan should include:

- <u>Tasks</u>: List all the tasks required to accomplish the goal.

- <u>Resources</u>: Identify the resources needed, such as tools, support, or information.

- <u>Deadlines</u>: Set deadlines for each task to ensure timely completion.

- <u>Responsibility</u>: Assign responsibilities if working in a team or if the goal involves multiple stakeholders.

Milestones

Milestones are significant checkpoints that mark progress towards the goal. Establish milestones to track achievements and make necessary adjustments. For example, if the goal is to write a book, milestones could include completing the outline, finishing the first draft, and finalizing the manuscript.

Action plans and milestones provide a clear roadmap for achieving goals, improve focus, and maintain motivation. They help in managing complex goals by breaking them into smaller, more manageable tasks and tracking progress systematically.

Tailor action plans and milestones to fit specific goals and personal preferences. Regularly review and update plans as progress is made or as circumstances change.

Overcoming Obstacles

Overcoming obstacles is a crucial aspect of achieving goals. We want to examine some common challenges faced during the goal-setting process and provide strategies for addressing and overcoming these obstacles.

Recognize potential challenges that may hinder progress, such as lack of resources, time constraints, or external factors. Understanding these obstacles helps in planning effective solutions.

Develop strategies to address challenges, including problem-solving techniques which involves developing solutions for identified challenges, seeking support from mentors, colleagues, or professional networks and adjusting goals or action plans in cases where unforeseen circumstances arise. Consider using resilience-building practices and maintaining a positive mindset.

Addressing obstacles proactively helps in maintaining momentum and achieving goals despite challenges. It encourages resilience and adaptability, ensuring that progress continues even when faced with setbacks.

Regularly assess potential obstacles and adjust strategies as needed. Stay proactive in seeking solutions and adapting plans to overcome challenges.

Review and Reflection

Regular review and reflection are essential for tracking progress and ensuring that goals are being met effectively.

Set regular intervals for reviewing progress towards goals. Evaluate whether tasks are being completed on time and if milestones are being achieved. Use this review process to identify any areas where adjustments are needed.

Reflect on the achievements, challenges faced, and lessons learned. Consider what worked well and what could be improved in future goal-setting efforts. Reflecting on the process helps in identifying strengths and areas for development.

Regular review and reflection provide insights into progress, help in making informed adjustments, and enhance the overall effectiveness of goal-setting strategies. It promotes continuous improvement and ensures that goals remain relevant and achievable.

Establish a review schedule that fits personal preferences and the nature of the goals. Use feedback from the review process to make informed adjustments and stay aligned with long-term objectives.

Applying these strategies for goal setting and achievement can effectively transform one's aspirations into actionable plans, enabling one to overcome obstacles, and stay motivated throughout the process.

PART 4: REAL-LIFE SUCCESS STORIES AND EXPERTS' INSIGHTS

Chapter 10

Inspiring Profiles of Success

There is a diverse collection of success stories from individuals who have effectively transformed stress and adversity into significant achievements. By examining these detailed profiles, you will gain insights into various fields, learn about the strategies employed, and understand the broader themes that contribute to success.

Diverse Fields of Achievement

First, we explore success stories across various domains such as business, sports, arts, and personal development. Each profile provides a comprehensive overview of the individual's background, the nature of their stress or adversity, and the paths they took to achieve success.

The Business Field

These profiles feature entrepreneurs who navigated financial crises, corporate leaders who turned challenges into growth opportunities, or innovators who leveraged stress to drive creative solutions.

One of such is Howard Schultz, the former CEO of Starbucks, who faced significant financial difficulties early in his career. After growing up in a poor neighborhood, he joined Starbucks when it was a small coffee bean retailer. Schultz envisioned transforming Starbucks into a coffeehouse experience and faced numerous challenges, including resistance from the company's original owners and securing funding. Despite these setbacks, Schultz's resilience and vision led him to create a global coffee empire. His ability to leverage stress into a drive for innovation and expansion exemplifies how overcoming adversity can lead to unprecedented success.

The Sports Domain

There are athletes who faced significant setbacks, such as injuries or intense competition, yet used these experiences to fuel their performance and achieve remarkable feats.

Serena Williams, a professional tennis player, is one athlete who faced significant stress and adversity throughout her career, including injuries and public scrutiny. Despite these challenges, Williams' dedication to training and her mental toughness allowed her to overcome setbacks and win multiple Grand Slam titles. Her ability to manage stress and maintain focus under pressure is a testament to her remarkable achievements and longevity in the sport.

Creative Arts

Even in the creative arts discipline, there are artists, writers, and performers who turned personal struggles into sources of inspiration and success, demonstrating how stress and adversity can enhance creativity and resilience.

J.K. Rowling, the author of the Harry Potter series, experienced profound personal difficulties, including poverty and rejection from publishers. Rowling's experience of hardship fueled her creativity, leading to the creation of one of the most beloved and successful literary franchises in history. Her story exemplifies how adversity can lead to groundbreaking success in the arts.

Personal Development

In the area of personal development, we have individuals who transformed their lives through personal growth, overcoming challenges such as health issues, or overcoming self-doubt to reach their goals.

Elizabeth Gilbert, author of "Eat, Pray, Love," faced a period of personal crisis following a divorce and professional burnout. Her journey of self-discovery and healing, documented in her memoir, inspired millions. Gilbert's story showcases how personal adversity can lead to profound personal growth and widespread influence.

Key Themes and Strategies

We can observe some common themes and strategies in these success stories. Patterns and approaches that contributed to overcoming adversity and achieving success can also be highlighted from these kinds of stories. Some of these include

Resilience and Adaptability

This examines how individuals demonstrated resilience by adapting to changing circumstances and using stress as a motivator for growth.

Jeff Bezos, the founder of Amazon, faced initial skepticism and numerous challenges when starting the company. He dealt with financial pressures, logistical issues, and competition. Bezos' resilience and willingness to adapt his business model, including moving from books to a wide range of products and embracing new technologies, were crucial in transforming Amazon into a global e-commerce leader.

Vision and Goal Setting

The importance of having a clear vision and setting specific goals that has guided individuals through their challenges and toward their achievements is another common theme and strategy.

Oprah Winfrey faced a challenging upbringing marked by poverty and abuse. Despite these difficulties, she maintained a clear vision of becoming a successful media personality. Winfrey set specific goals, such as becoming a news anchor, which led her to eventually create a highly successful talk show and media empire. Her ability to set and pursue her goals through periods of significant stress is a testament to the power of vision and goal-setting.

Support Systems

The role of mentors, coaches, family, or networks in providing support, guidance, and motivation during times of stress can also be observed to be a very important theme

Steve Jobs, co-founder of Apple Inc., experienced significant stress during his career, including being ousted from the company he founded. During this period, Jobs received crucial support from friends and mentors, including Pixar's CEO, Ed Catmull. This support system helped Jobs to not only overcome his challenges but also return to Apple and lead it to unprecedented success. Jobs' story underscores the importance of having a strong support network during stressful times.

Learning and Growth

Individuals turned their experiences of stress and failure into opportunities for learning and personal development.

Nelson Mandela spent 27 years in prison under harsh conditions. Despite the immense stress and adversity, Mandela used his time in prison for personal growth and to develop a vision for a post-apartheid South Africa. Upon his release, he successfully led negotiations to end apartheid and became the country's first Black president. Mandela's experience illustrates how adversity and stress can be used as a foundation for significant personal and societal change.

Lessons Learned

Finally, we distill the key lessons and insights from the profiles and themes discussed. These lessons serve as actionable takeaways to apply to your own life.

Applying Strategies

This success story presents practical advice on how to use the strategies we have observed to address personal challenges and goals.

Angela Duckworth, a psychologist and author of "Grit," used her own experiences of overcoming academic and professional challenges to develop her theory of grit. Duckworth's strategies for applying perseverance and passion to long-term goals are drawn from her personal journey of facing setbacks and using them to fuel her success. Her work provides actionable advice on how to apply resilience and perseverance in one's own life.

Overcoming Adversity

This story gives insights into how stress can be reframed as a source of strength and opportunity, rather than merely a barrier.

Malala Yousafzai, Pakistani activist for female education, survived an assassination attempt by the Taliban due to her activism. Her ability to turn this traumatic experience into a global platform for advocating education and women's rights demonstrates how extreme adversity can be transformed into a force for widespread positive change. Yousafzai's story serves as an example of how one can overcome significant challenges and use them to inspire and enact meaningful change.

Inspiration and Motivation

Finally, an encouragement for you to draw inspiration from the success stories and recognize your own potential for achieving remarkable outcomes despite stress.

Nick Vujicic, born without arms or legs, faced significant personal and societal challenges. His ability to overcome these challenges and become a renowned motivational speaker exemplifies how personal adversity can be turned into a source of inspiration for others. Vujicic's story encourages readers to see their own struggles as opportunities for growth and to find motivation in the face of adversity.

These examples illustrate the diverse ways in which individuals from various fields have transformed stress and adversity into significant achievements, offering valuable lessons and motivation for readers.

Chapter 11

First-hand Insights from Experts and Achievers

Insights from Dr. Martin Seligman

Dr. Martin Seligman on Positive Psychology and how positive psychology techniques can help individuals manage stress.

Dr. Martin Seligman, a leading figure in positive psychology shared his expert views on how his field provides effective strategies for managing stress. He emphasized the importance of focusing on well-being by leveraging individual strengths and fostering positive emotions. Dr. Seligman highlighted the practice of gratitude as a powerful tool in stress management. By regularly acknowledging and appreciating positive experiences, individuals can shift their focus away from stressors, thereby building resilience. He mentioned that keeping a gratitude journal, where one records daily positive moments, can significantly counteract stress.

Dr. Seligman also discussed resilience training, noting that it involves developing the ability to bounce back from adversity. He suggested that cognitive-behavioral techniques, such as cognitive restructuring, are effective in helping individuals reframe their thinking and approach challenges with a growth mindset. Viewing setbacks as learning opportunities rather than failures can enhance resilience and transform stress into a tool for personal growth.

Perspectives from Dr. Brene Brown

Dr. Brene Brown on Vulnerability and Empathy and how they help with stress handling and management

Dr. Brene Brown, renowned for her research on Vulnerability and Empathy, shared insights on how these concepts play crucial roles in stress management. According to Dr. Brown, embracing vulnerability allows individuals to be authentic and build deeper connections with others, which can alleviate stress. By sharing struggles with trusted friends or colleagues, people can foster supportive relationships that reduce feelings of isolation.

Dr. Brown also discussed the significance of empathy. She explained that practicing empathy helps individuals connect with others on a deeper level, which in turn provides a sense of belonging and support. This connection can be particularly valuable in stressful situations, as empathetic interactions can lessen the emotional burden. Simple acts of listening and understanding are highlighted as impactful ways to manage stress.

Reflections from Elon Musk

Elon Musk on managing stress in high-pressure environments and strategies for handling setbacks and failures

Elon Musk, CEO of Tesla, known for his intense work ethic and high-pressure roles, described his approach to stress management through structured strategies like time blocking. By allocating specific time slots for different tasks, Musk is able to focus intensely on one task at a time, which helps manage stress and improve productivity. This method involves creating a structured approach to tackle complex problems without feeling overwhelmed.

Musk also addressed how he handles failure and setbacks, viewing them as integral parts of the learning process. He analyzes what went wrong and seeks to understand how to improve, which helps transform setbacks into opportunities for growth rather than sources of discouragement. His advice for managing stress in high-pressure environments includes developing a structured task approach and maintaining a resilience mindset.

Reflections from Oprah Winfrey

Oprah Winfrey on self-care and emotional resilience as effective and proven personal practices for managing stress

Oprah Winfrey, known for her focus on self-care and balance, shared how these practices are integral to managing stress. She highlighted the importance of incorporating self-care routines, such as meditation, exercise, and a balanced diet, into daily life. Starting her day with meditation, for instance, helps her maintain a positive mindset and manage stress effectively

She also touched on emotional resilience, highlighting the importance of maintaining a positive outlook and practicing mindfulness. Techniques such as affirmations and mindfulness help her stay focused and balanced, contributing to effective stress management. Winfrey suggested incorporating small self-care activities into daily routines, such as meditation and physical activity, to make a significant difference in managing stress and maintaining well-being.

Cross-Disciplinary Views

Insights from Satya Nadella

Satya Nadella on how psychological principles influence leadership approach

Satya Nadella, CEO of Microsoft, discussed the significant role of psychological principles in his leadership approach. He explained that integrating stress management strategies, such as regular feedback sessions and emotional intelligence training, is fundamental to fostering a positive organizational culture. These practices support employee well-being and contribute to a more engaged and productive workforce.

Nadella elaborated on how prioritizing emotional intelligence and creating an open feedback environment enhances leadership effectiveness. The focus on developing empathy and resilience in leadership training helps leaders manage their own stress while better supporting their teams. This approach not only improves individual performance but also strengthens the overall organizational climate.

Reflections from Michael Phelps

Michael Phelps on his approach to stress management and the techniques he has found most effective

Michael Phelps, a celebrated Olympian, shared his approach to stress management, which includes visualization and goal setting as key techniques. He described how visualizing every aspect of a race helps him prepare both physically and mentally, significantly reducing performance anxiety. Setting clear goals is another strategy he employs to maintain focus and manage stress effectively.

Phelps extended these techniques beyond the swimming pool, noting their applicability to various life areas. Whether facing personal or professional challenges, he uses visualization and goal setting to stay mentally prepared and focused. This approach involves maintaining a clear vision and taking actionable steps toward achieving one's goals, demonstrating how these principles can be valuable in diverse contexts.

Chapter 12

Applying Success Stories to Everyday Life

Success stories provide not only inspiration but also practical lessons that can be directly applied to our own lives. By examining how successful individuals navigate their challenges, we gain valuable insights that can be adapted to our personal journeys.

Practical Lessons for Daily Living

Adopting a Growth Mindset

Consider Oprah Winfrey, whose rise from overcoming significant personal and professional obstacles to becoming a global icon exemplifies the power of a growth mindset. Winfrey's ability to view her setbacks as opportunities for learning and growth allowed her to transform adversity into a catalyst for her success.

This approach teaches us the importance of adopting a growth mindset ourselves. When faced with challenges, we should focus on what we can learn from each experience and how it can contribute to our personal development.

Implementing Structured Planning

Elon Musk's methodical approach to managing multiple high-profile ventures offers another useful lesson. Musk utilizes rigorous time management techniques and task prioritization to effectively handle complex projects and high-pressure situations.

His use of time blocking and systematic problem-solving provides a model for enhancing productivity and reducing stress. To adapt this to our own lives, we can develop a structured plan for our tasks and goals. Implementing techniques like time blocking helps manage our workload and reduce feelings of overwhelm.

Practicing Resilience and Adaptability

Dr. Martin Seligman's research on resilience underscores the value of cognitive restructuring and resilience training in overcoming adversity. Seligman's principles highlight that resilience is crucial for managing stress effectively.

By practicing cognitive restructuring—reframing negative thoughts and focusing on positive aspects—we can build our resilience and better handle stress. This involves viewing challenges as opportunities for growth and adapting our strategies to overcome obstacles.

Adapting Strategies

Adapting strategies from success stories involves tailoring techniques and insights to fit individual needs and contexts. Here are ways to adapt the strategies discussed:

To integrate these insights into our lives, we first need to personalize our approach. Applying SMART goals—Specific, Measurable, Achievable, Relevant, Time-bound—can help us set clear, actionable objectives. Breaking down long-term goals into smaller, manageable steps and regularly reviewing and adjusting these goals ensures they remain aligned with our priorities and circumstances.

Incorporating self-care practices is another crucial aspect. Oprah Winfrey's routine, which includes meditation and regular exercise, serves as a reminder of the importance of self-care. By identifying activities that resonate with us, such as mindfulness practices or physical exercise, and incorporating them into our daily routine, we can support our overall well-being and manage stress more effectively.

Emotional intelligence plays a significant role in managing stress and building supportive relationships. Brene Brown's emphasis on vulnerability and empathy illustrates how emotional intelligence can enhance our interactions and resilience. To leverage this, we should practice empathy and active listening in our interactions, develop self-awareness, and regulate our emotions. This approach not only supports our emotional resilience but also strengthens our interpersonal relationships.

Inspiring Action

Applying the lessons from success stories can inspire actionable steps for personal and professional growth. Here's how to translate inspiration into concrete actions:

1. Create a Personal Action Plan

Turning these lessons into actionable steps involves creating a detailed personal action plan. For instance, if we are inspired by Elon Musk's time management techniques, we might develop a daily or weekly schedule that incorporates time blocking and task prioritization.

2. Establish Support Networks

Establishing support networks is another key action. Building relationships with professionals and peers who share similar goals can provide valuable support and insights.

3. Reflect and Adjust Regularly

Finally, regular reflection and adjustment are vital. Using tools like journaling or self-assessment, we can evaluate our progress and make necessary adjustments to stay aligned with our goals.

By applying these actionable takeaways, adapting strategies to fit our personal contexts, and taking inspired actions, we can effectively incorporate lessons from success stories into our own lives.

PART 5:
HOLISTIC APPROACHES TO STRESS AND WELL-BEING

Chapter 13

Integrating Stress Management with Wellness Practices

In the quest for effective stress management, incorporating comprehensive wellness practices is essential. This chapter delves into how integrating exercise, nutrition, sleep, and balanced routines can enhance overall well-being and help manage stress more effectively.

The Role of Exercise

Exercise is a cornerstone of stress management. Engaging in physical activity triggers the release of endorphins, the body's natural mood lifters, and helps lower cortisol levels, the stress hormone. Regular exercise, including aerobic activities such as running, swimming, and biking, as well as strength training and flexibility exercises like yoga, offers profound benefits for both mental and physical health.

Studies underscore the value of exercise in stress reduction. For instance, research published in the "Journal of Clinical Psychiatry" highlights that individuals who maintain a regular exercise regimen report significantly lower levels of anxiety and depression. Exercise not only improves sleep quality and boosts self-esteem but also fosters resilience against stress.

Incorporating Exercise into Daily Life

To reap the benefits of exercise, start by finding activities that you genuinely enjoy. Whether it's dancing, hiking, or playing a sport, engaging in enjoyable activities makes exercise a more pleasant and sustainable part of your routine.

Set realistic and attainable goals—begin with 20-minute sessions three times a week and gradually increase both the frequency and duration of your workouts. Consistency is crucial, so schedule your workouts like any other important appointment.

Nutritional Strategies

Nutrition is another vital aspect of stress management. A balanced diet provides essential nutrients that support brain function and mood stabilization. Foods rich in omega-3 fatty acids, such as salmon and flaxseeds, and those high in antioxidants, like berries and leafy greens, help reduce inflammation and improve mental clarity.

Key Nutritional Components for Stress Management

Incorporate complex carbohydrates, like whole grains and legumes, into your diet to stabilize blood sugar levels, which helps prevent mood swings and irritability. Lean proteins, including chicken and tofu, support neurotransmitter function, crucial for mood regulation. Adequate hydration is equally important; dehydration can exacerbate stress and fatigue, so aim to drink plenty of water throughout the day.

Practical Tips for Healthy Eating

Plan your meals in advance to ensure you have nutritious options readily available and reduce the temptation to choose unhealthy foods. Practice mindful eating by paying attention to hunger and fullness cues and eating slowly to savor your food. Limit caffeine and sugar intake, as excessive consumption can lead to energy crashes and heightened stress. Opt for balanced meals and snacks that provide sustained energy.

Importance of Sleep

Sleep plays a critical role in managing stress. Poor sleep can negatively affect mood, cognitive function, and overall health. Quality sleep helps regulate stress hormones and supports emotional resilience. Establishing a regular sleep routine—going to bed and waking up at the same time each day—can significantly improve sleep quality and make falling asleep easier.

Strategies for Improving Sleep Quality

Create a relaxing bedtime routine to signal to your body that it's time to wind down. Engage in calming activities such as reading or practicing mindfulness before bed. Optimize your sleep environment by ensuring your bedroom is cool, dark, and quiet, and invest in a comfortable mattress and pillows to support restful sleep.

Creating a Balanced Routine

A balanced daily routine that integrates exercise, nutrition, and sleep is essential for managing stress effectively. Schedule dedicated time for self-care activities, including exercise, meal preparation, and relaxation. Define clear boundaries between work and personal time to avoid overworking and ensure you have ample time for rest and leisure.

Practical Tips for a Balanced Routine

Allocate specific times for self-care activities and stick to them. Flexibility is important, so adapt your routine as needed while maintaining a focus on overall well-being. By prioritizing these wellness practices, you build a robust foundation for managing stress and leading a healthier, more fulfilling life.

Chapter 14

Achieving Work-Life Balance

Work-life balance is a crucial component of effective stress management and overall well-being. Here, we explore what constitutes work-life balance, strategies for achieving it, methods for avoiding burnout, and real-life success stories that illustrate these concepts.

Work-Life Balance and Burnout

Work-life balance involves managing professional and personal responsibilities in a way that promotes health, productivity, and satisfaction in both areas. It is not a static state but a dynamic process of adjusting priorities based on changing circumstances and needs. Achieving work-life balance means creating boundaries that protect personal time and ensuring that work demands do not overwhelm one's personal life.

Burnout is a state of chronic physical and emotional exhaustion often caused by prolonged stress and overwork. It manifests as feelings of fatigue, decreased performance, and detachment from work.

Strategies for Balance

The strategies for achieving work-life balance includes:

1. Setting Boundaries

One of the foundational strategies for achieving work-life balance is setting clear boundaries between work and personal life. This involves defining specific work hours and adhering to them as strictly as possible. For instance, setting a firm end time for the workday and avoiding work-related tasks during personal time can help create a clear separation.

2. Prioritizing Tasks

Effective time management involves prioritizing tasks based on their urgency and importance. Tools such as the Eisenhower Matrix can help categorize tasks into four quadrants—urgent and important, important but not urgent, urgent but not important, and neither urgent nor important. This categorization helps focus efforts on high-priority tasks and delegate or defer less critical ones.

3. Implementing Flexibility

Flexibility in work arrangements, such as telecommuting or flexible hours, can significantly contribute to work-life balance. This flexibility allows individuals to adapt their work schedules to better accommodate personal responsibilities and preferences, reducing stress and improving job satisfaction.

4. Practicing Self-Care

Self-care is essential for maintaining balance and preventing burnout. Incorporating regular physical activity, relaxation techniques, and hobbies into one's routine helps manage stress and rejuvenate the mind and body. Activities such as meditation, reading, or spending time with loved ones can provide essential breaks from work-related stressors.

Avoiding Burnout

Avoiding burnout involves recognizing its signs early and taking proactive steps to address them.

1. Recognizing Signs of Burnout

Common signs of burnout include persistent tiredness, irritability, reduced productivity, and a sense of disconnection from work. Monitoring these signs and being aware of their impact on both mental and physical health is crucial for timely intervention.

2. Seeking Support

Seeking support from supervisors, colleagues, or mental health professionals can help address burnout. Open communication about workload and stress levels with supervisors can lead to adjustments in responsibilities or additional resources to alleviate pressure.

3. Taking Regular Breaks

Scheduled breaks during work hours are vital for maintaining productivity and preventing burnout. Short breaks for physical movement, stretching, or brief mental relaxation can help refresh the mind and body, improving focus and reducing stress.

Conclusion

Summary of Key Points

In this book, we have embarked on a transformative journey to redefine our relationship with stress and anxiety. We began by exploring the nature of stress and its impact on our lives, delving into the mind-body connection and the scientific principles that underpin these experiences. We examined how reframing adversity can turn challenges into opportunities for personal growth, and we applied psychological theories and principles of positive psychology to enhance our resilience.

We then moved to practical strategies and tools, providing actionable techniques such as cognitive restructuring, journaling, and productivity hacks. These tools are designed to manage stress effectively while improving overall productivity. Through personal stories and case studies, we drew inspiration from individuals who have successfully harnessed stress to achieve their goals. Lastly, we integrated holistic approaches, emphasizing the importance of exercise, nutrition, and work-life balance in maintaining long-term wellness and resilience.

Commitment to the Journey

As you close this book, remember that transforming stress into a powerful force for personal growth requires commitment and persistence. The techniques and insights provided are not merely theoretical; they are practical steps that can lead to profound changes in your life. Embrace these strategies with an open mind and heart, and be patient with yourself as you implement them. The journey towards harnessing the positives of stress is ongoing, and the benefits will become evident as you persist and apply what you've learned. Trust the process, stay committed to your personal growth, and allow yourself to experience the transformative effects of these practices.

Final Thoughts

In the end, "Turning Stress and Anxiety Around" is more than just a guide—it's an invitation to reclaim your power and redefine your relationship with stress. By shifting your perspective and embracing the principles outlined in this book, you are not only managing stress but also using it as a catalyst for growth and achievement. Life's challenges are inevitable, but how you respond to them can make all the difference.

Remember that every setback is an opportunity for a comeback, and every challenge is a chance to grow stronger and wiser. As you move forward, may you find strength in adversity, wisdom in your experiences, and fulfillment in your journey toward a balanced and successful life.